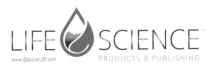

www.DiscoverLSP.com

PRODUCTS & PUBLISHING

Copyright © 2018
Life Science Publishing
1.800.336.6308
www.DiscoverLSP.com

Printed in the United States of America
10 9 8 7 6 5 4 3 2 1

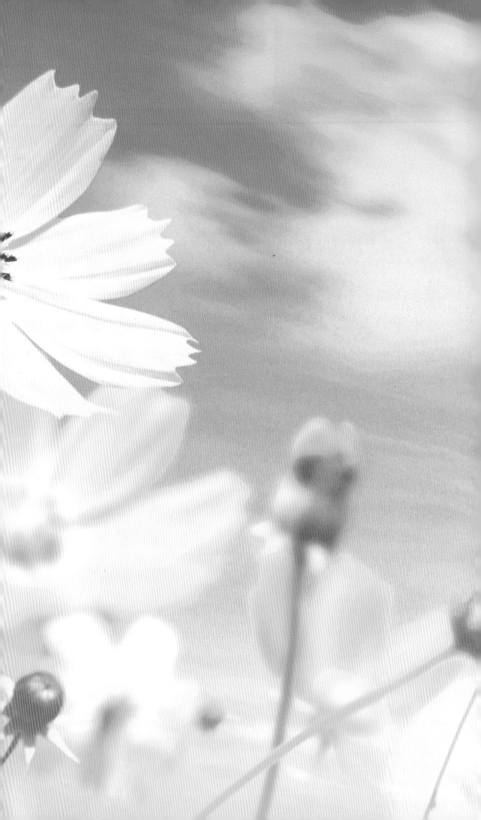

Table of Contents

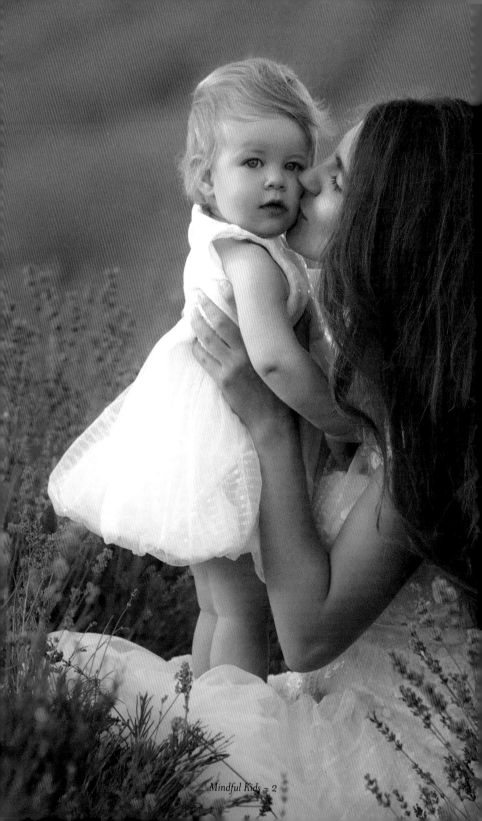

"Smell is a potent wizard that transports you across thousands of miles and all the years you have lived."
— Helen Keller

Young Living Loves Our Trees

The smell of Einkorn pancakes filled the air as we prepared to plant the Idaho Balsam Fir saplings. The weather was cold, with drizzle turning to sleet, offering us moisture to naturally water our babies and soften the soil for planting. We first mapped out the land with rope and sticks to set our rows vertically and horizontally. Then Gary Young taught us how to plant. There were 23 of us from all around the globe coming together to be stewards of the land in Young Living fashion. Young Living is a protector of our earth, the trees, plants, and all living things.

The air was fresh as we were breathing in the oxygen from the grandmother/father balsam fir trees surrounding our planting zones. It was nice to be on the land with our hands in the dirt digging 6-inch holes for new balsam saplings. For every tree harvested to distill our Idaho Balsam Fir essential oil, two more trees are planted to restore the forest. In Idaho, our farms are full of Idaho Balsam Fir trees that are elderly and ready to harvest. In the land where we harvest, we restore with our reforestation projects during Spring planting time. Our efforts supporting the reforestation project plan of planting 5000 Idaho Balsam Fir trees in two weeks, contributed to the cycle of photosynthesis.

Young Living loves our trees. Trees and humans thrive off one another. The trees turn carbon dioxide into oxygen for us to breathe. Every time a human and/or animal breathes, we turn oxygen into carbon dioxide for the trees to absorb. This is an even exchange and continuous flow of life energy between trees and humans. Everyone could FEEL the life energy all around us. This planting experience was a true testament to the environmental elements supporting the life energy of our essential oils.

While we were in this field, it was sunny, rainy, cold, warm, wet, dry, and earthy. The environment shifted and changed hourly and sometimes moment to moment. I became so overjoyed with the aroma of the balsam fir I felt the need to pay homage to the trees standing tall. I ran to the edge of the open field where we were surrounded by the tallest of trees. I hugged those grandparents surrounding us saying Thank You for their gifts – oxygen, protection, aroma, and essential oils.

There is nothing more humbling than spending time on our Young Living farms and serving our Earth. This is the foundation of what Young Living is all about. Our farms offering us pure, therapeutic essential oils is a gift provided to us by our founder, Mary & Gary Young and Mother Earth. We thank you for these gifts!

The Inspiration for the ABC's & Essential Oils

The ABC's and Young Living Essential Oils are the perfect combination to instill creative learning, wonder, and imagination within our children. The letters and sounds of the alphabet are the building blocks of the English language, as the elements of carbon, hydrogen, and oxygen are the building blocks of life on earth. The essential elements of carbon, hydrogen, and oxygen inherent in the bark, leaves, stems, plants, roots, and flowers distilled to create Young Living Essential Oils contain the key to integrate and learn the ABC's. Discover the connection with your children on the alphabet adventure.

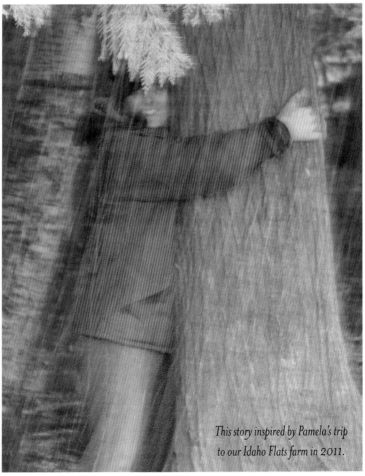

This story inspired by Pamela's trip to our Idaho Flats farm in 2011.

Mindful Kids

Yoga means union. Yoga brings together our body, breath, and mind. Practicing kid's yoga is all about awareness – in your body and the world around you. Kids naturally reflect the world around them imitating animals, sounds, trees, mountains, stars, etc. In kid's yoga, we practice mindful movements to bring awareness to their natural reflections.

What are Essential Oils?

Essential Oils are liquids that easily evaporate in the air and absorb into the skin. They are distilled from roots, stems, leaves, flowers, bark or resin of plants. They are the life energy of the plant kingdom. This life energy extends the wellness and life of the plant.

▶Dakota (9-years-old) asks, *"Is this life energy in my body?"*

We reply, *"Yes! We are made of the same elements - carbon, hydrogen, and oxygen. We have a unique connection with plants. We need each other. We can easily absorb essential oils into our bodies because we are made of the same stuff. We give each other life energy! Let us explain more...."*

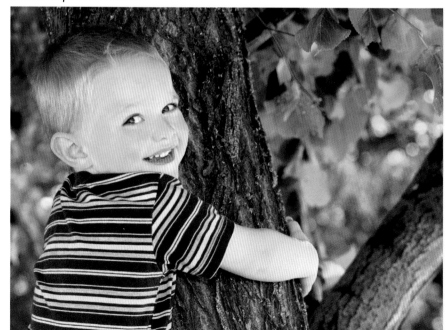

Carbon is one of the most important elements. It is the building block of life and the second most abundant element in the human body making up 18 percent. Plants obtain carbon from the atmosphere, humans, and animals through the process of photosynthesis much like humans receive carbon dioxide.

Hydrogen is the lightest of the elements and the most abundant in the Universe. The most common place we find hydrogen is in water. It is also abundant in the stars! Ninety percent of all the atoms in the Universe are hydrogen with 10% of the human body being hydrogen.

Oxygen is the most important element needed on earth for life to survive! It is the 3rd most abundant element in the Universe, but the MOST abundant in the human body – 65%! Plants create the majority of the oxygen we breathe through photosynthesis.

▶ Dakota expresses,
   "That is so cool. Humans and essential oils are so connected!"

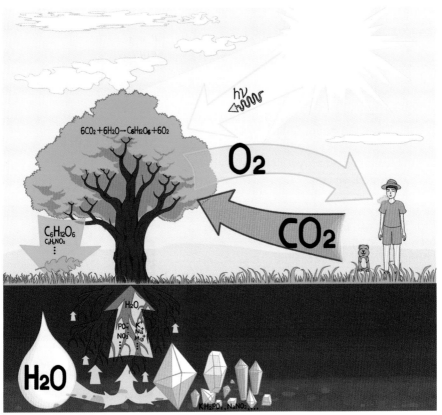

Essential Oils with Kids

To introduce kids to essential oils, we recommend starting with familiar scents first, such as citrus, floral, or woodsy aromas. Be playful and mindful with your kids by bringing them into the process of learning and discovering essential oils.

We will be using two methods of application – inhalation and topical.

Inhalation Method

A subtle way to offer essential oils to your kids is to wave the cap of the essential oil bottle under their nose rather than have them hold the bottle and smell it themselves. This is a very safe way to introduce oils and allows them to smell the scent with less potency. Simply breathing in essential oils is amazing and effective! The sense of smell is the only sense that travels directly to the brain. The essential oil aroma travels through the olfactory bulb to the Limbic brain where memory and emotions are stored.

Ways to use the inhalation method:
- Smelling the cap of the bottle or directly from the bottle.
- Diffusing with water or with a waterless diffuser.
- Placing 1-2 drops on a cotton pad (can easily be removed from an area).
- Scent Tent – dropping 1-3 drops in the palm of your hands, rubbing your hands together clockwise 3x and placing your palms over your nose like a 'tent' to breathe in the aroma.

SCENT TENT

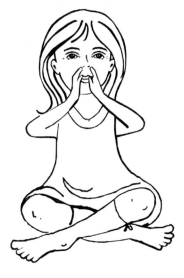

Kids are drawn to what they need. Often, they walk up to your oil collection and choose what oils attract them. It is so fun to see what they choose!

The intelligence of essential oils is fascinating! For kids, when applying topically, it is recommended to dilute with a carrier oil for kids under 5 years of age. The bottom of the feet is said to be the safest place to apply topically. The essential oils have their own intelligence and travel where they are needed in the body.

Basic Guidelines for Safe Use

STORAGE	CAUTIONARY USE	Application
Store in amber bottles	Oils rich in menthol (peppermint) are not suggested to be used on neck or throat area of children < 18 months	Topically apply oils to bottoms of feet or use in bath water, no more than 10 drops
Capped tightly	Citrus oils, Bergamot are photosensitive. Stay out of sun, 1-2 days after application or cover usage area.	Direct inhalation of oils, up to 10-15 times daily
Keep in cool location, out of light	Keep essential oils from eyes and ears. Do not touch eyes, glasses, or contact lenses.	Inhalation of oils not recommended for asthmatics
Keep out of reach of children	People exhibiting chronic, pre-existing health conditions (epilepsy, hypertension, i.e.) should consult physician before use. Particular caution with high ketone oils such as, Basil, Rosemary, Sage, and Tansy oils.	Before internal ingestion, try dilution in Blue Agave, Yacon syrups, or olive or coconut oils, rice milk
Keep vegetable oil on hand for dilution (V-6 Oil complex, other veggie oils)	Pregnant women or people exhibiting allergies should consult their physicians prior to use. Dilution of oils with a vegetable-based oil suggested. Skin patch test on the underside of the arm for 30 minutes warranted. Use common sense.	Reactions to essential oils, topically or by ingestion, may be delayed 2-3 days after use

8 Tips for Oily Yoga Play

1. Plan quality time with your kids to explore movement and essential oils in a playful setting.

2. Turn off electronics and be present with each other.

3. Gather your Young Living Essential Oils referenced in this book and/or your favorites.

4. Find an indoor or outdoor spacious area to move freely.

5. Hold hands and say the **Mindful Kids Pledge.** (page 12)

6. If it's your first time with this book, start at letter "A" and begin your Affirmation Alphabet Adventure.

7. Practice and play regularly.

8. This is a wonderful time to use **positive reinforcement.** (page 45)

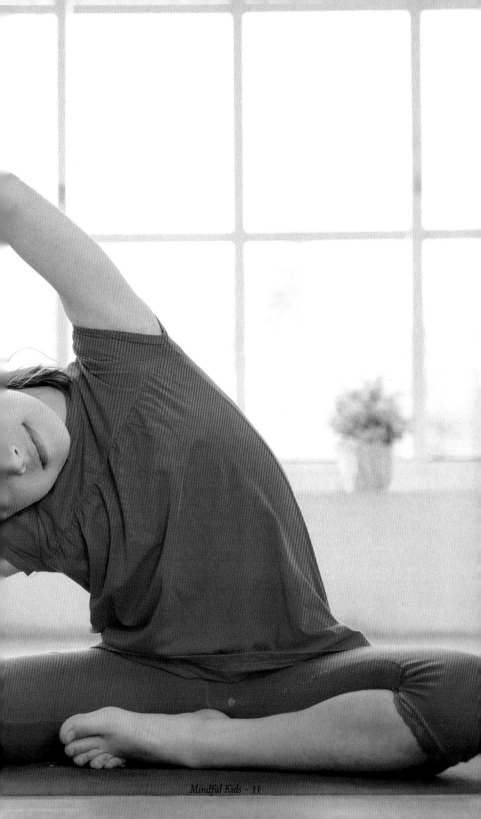

Mindful Kids Pledge

I connect to the life energy in our planet.
I am alive.
I connect to the life energy in our essential oils.
I am healthy.
I connect to the life energy in my body.
I am radiant.
I connect to the life energy in my family.
I am love.
I move freely, live joyfully, and love fully.

Yoga Affirmation ABCs & Essential Oils Adventure

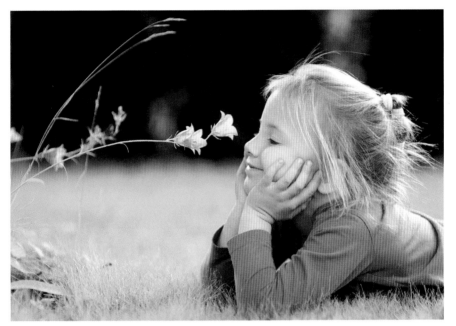

- Open your oil bottle and breathe in the aroma using the inhalation method.
- Stand in Mountain Pose
- Make the letter on the page with your body
- Say the affirmation out loud 3x
  One time for your body, one time for you mind, one time for your heart!
- Inhale your essential oil with your 'scent tent' (page 8) or open bottle
- Breathe in the oil 3x
  One time for your body, one time for you mind, one time for your heart!

Move throughout the entire alphabet, one letter at a time, and get acquainted with all the letters. Start simple for children learning the alphabet. Do not attempt to teach all 26 letters at once. Simply concentrate on a few letters at a time and allow your child to see, hear, and experience that letter in a variety of ways as guided in our book. The most important teaching tip of all is to make it fun. Make it a game and your child will love learning with you.

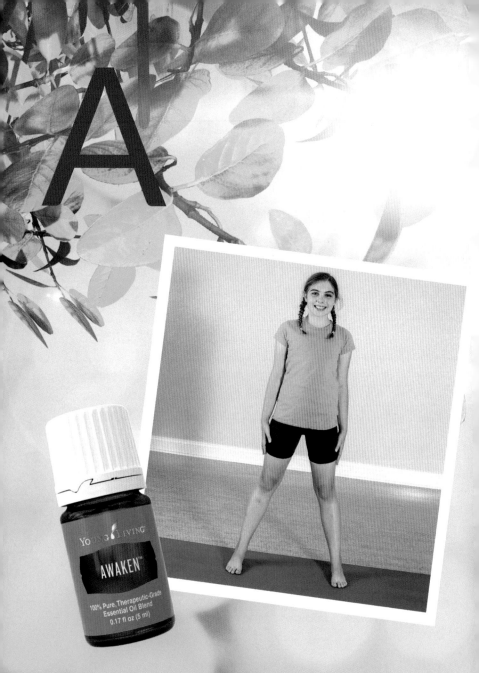

A

I awaken my energy.

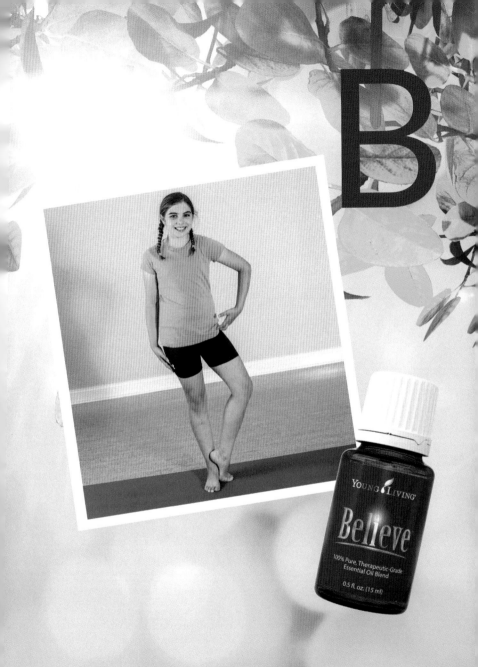

I believe in myself.

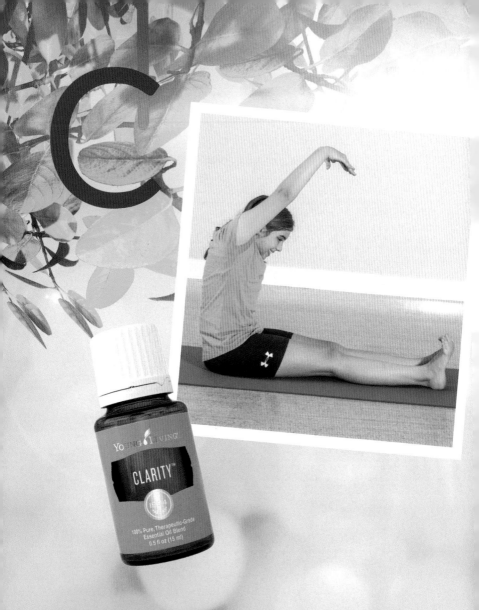

I have clarity.

D

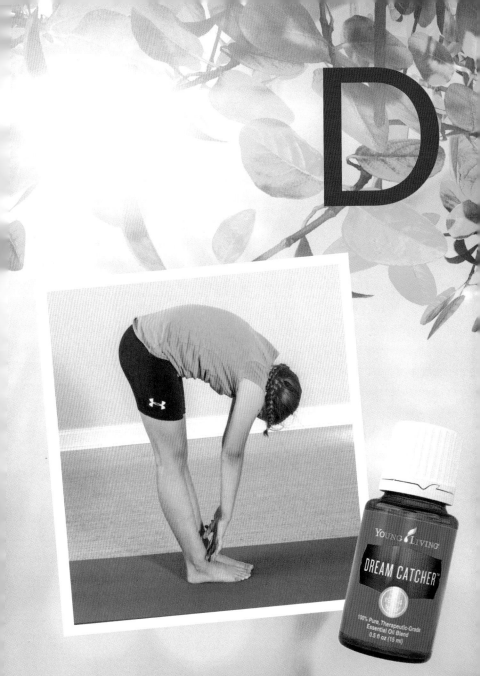

I am dreaming big!

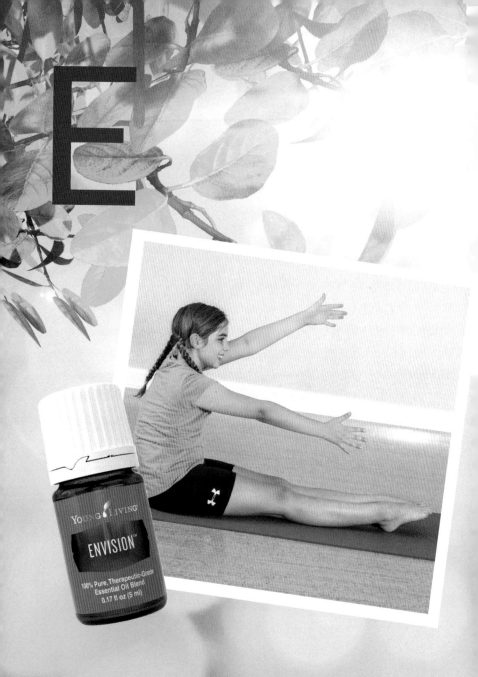

E

I envision my day.

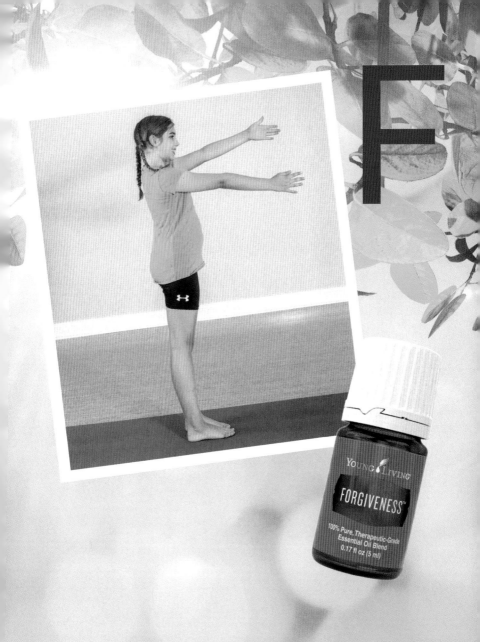

F

I choose forgiveness.

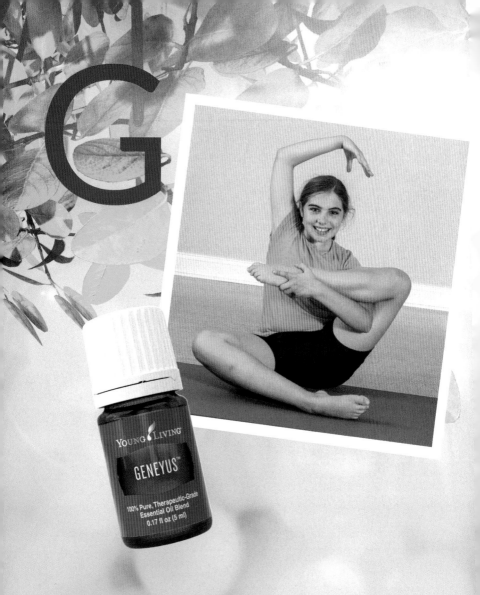

G

GENEYUS

I am a genius.

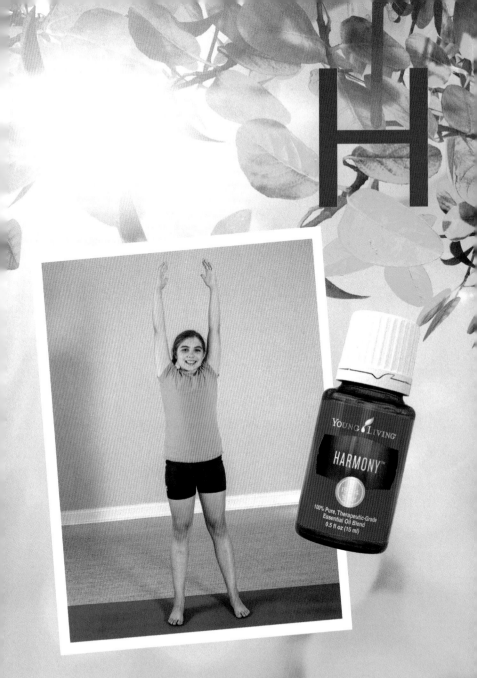

I live in harmony.

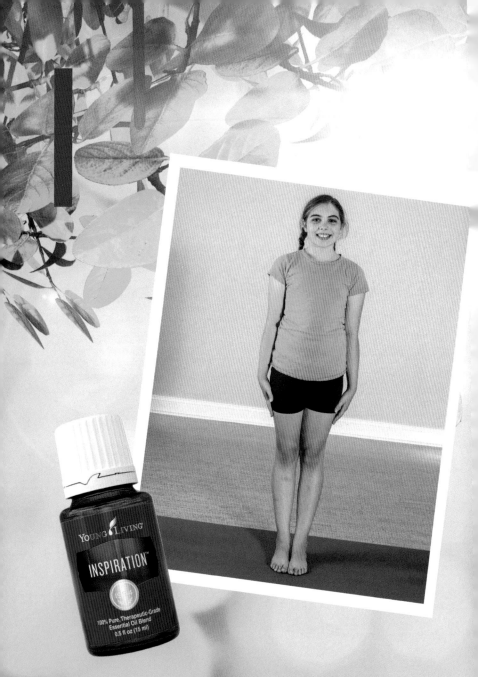

I receive inspiration.

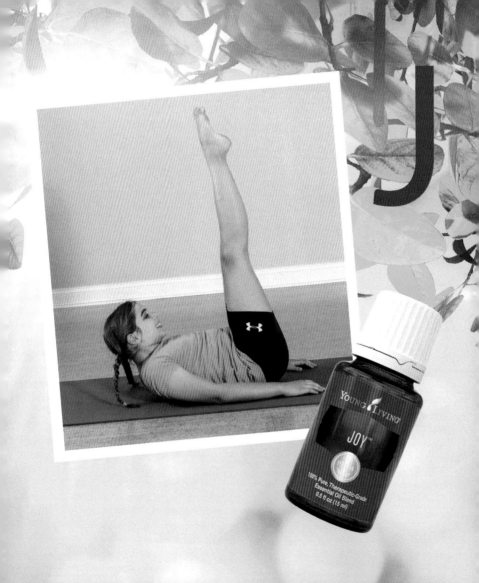

I love joy.

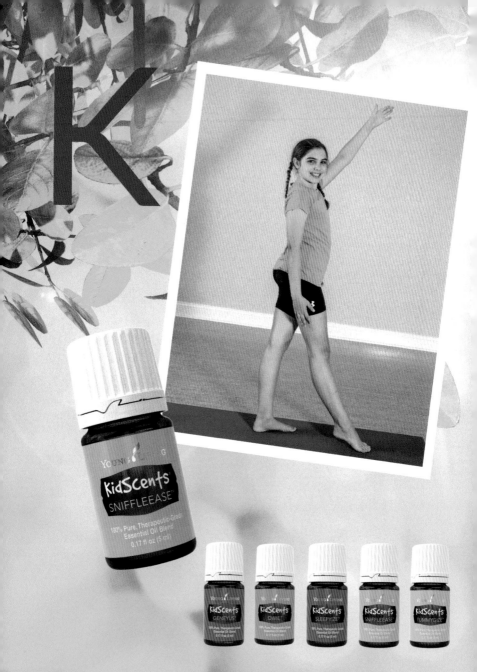

I enjoy Kidscents oils.

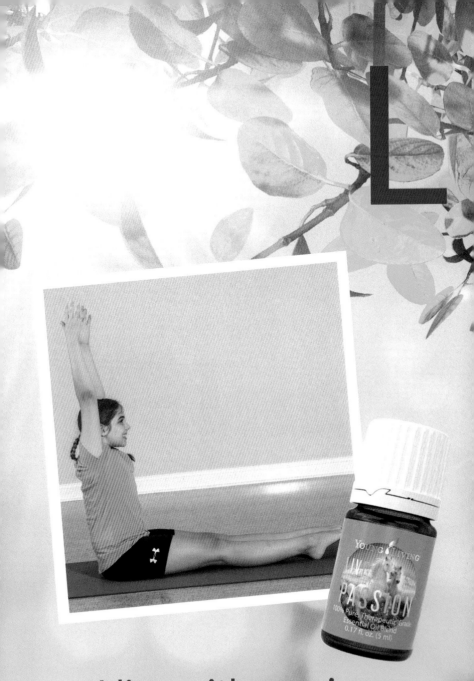

I live with passion.

M

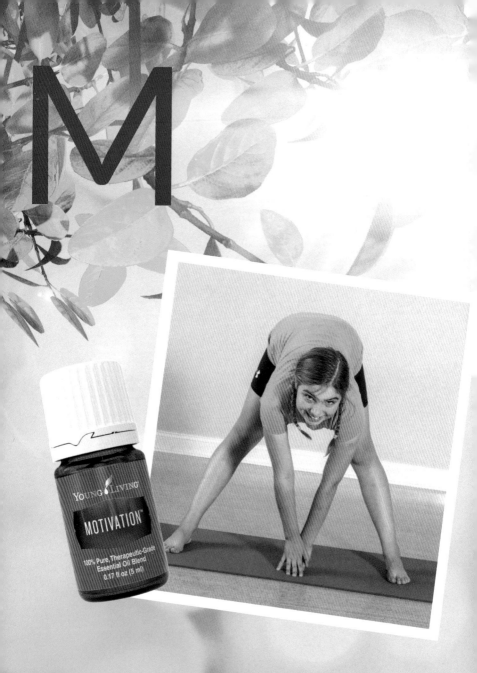

MOTIVATION™

100% Pure, Therapeutic-Grade
Essential Oil Blend
0.17 fl oz (5 ml)

I have motivation.

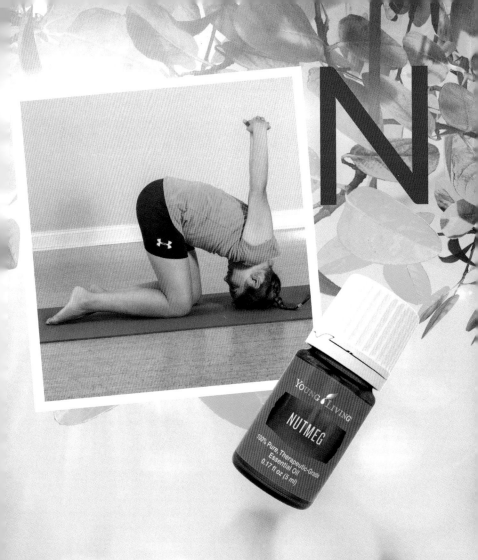

I am inhaling
nutmeg to relax.

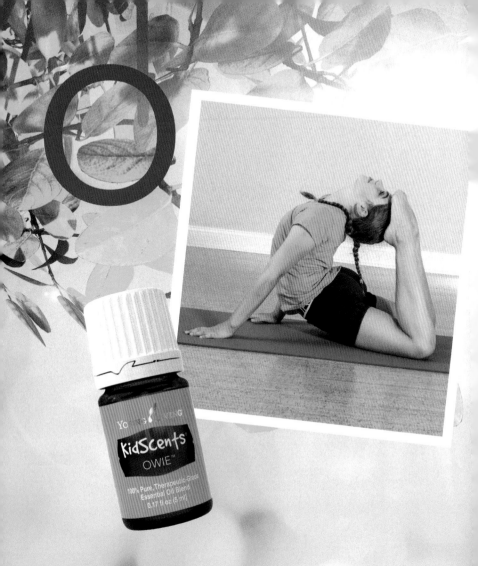

No more owies for me!

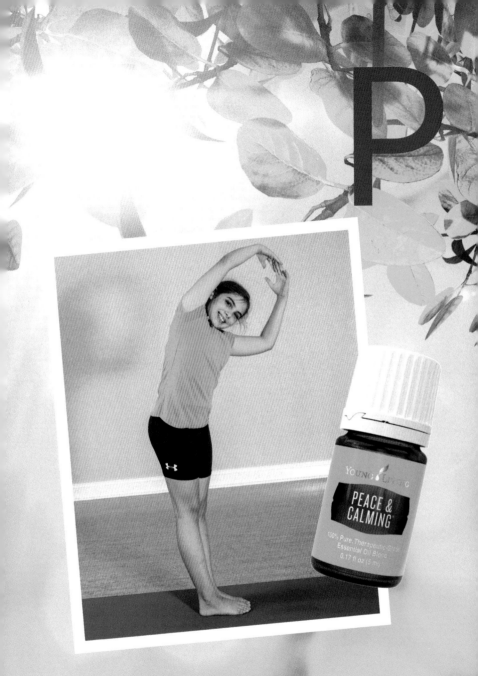

I feel peace and calm.

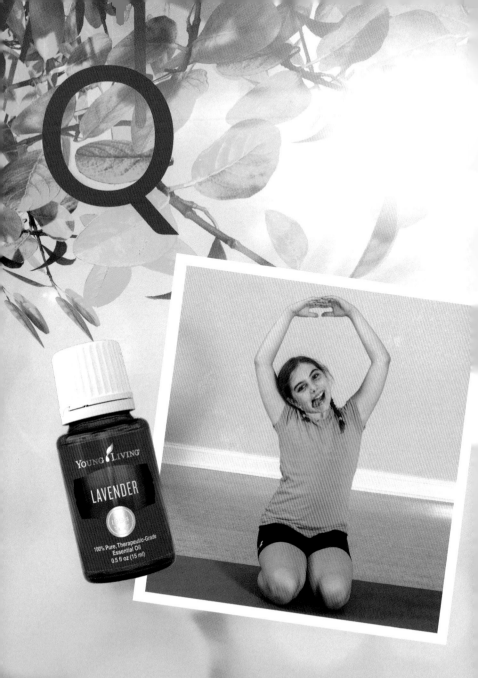

Quiet time with lavender. I love lavender.

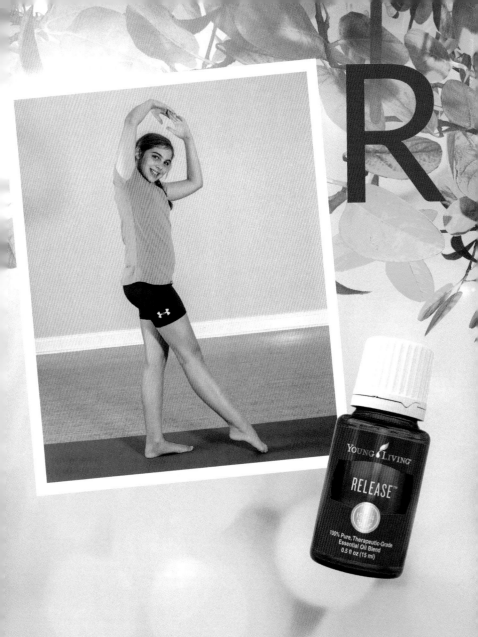

I release my anger gently.

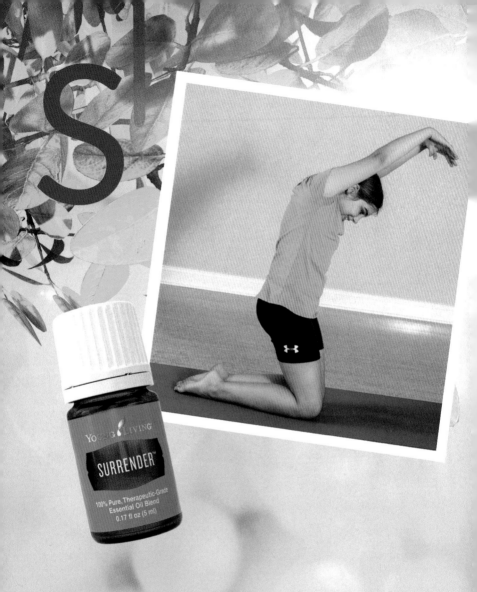

S

I choose to surrender.

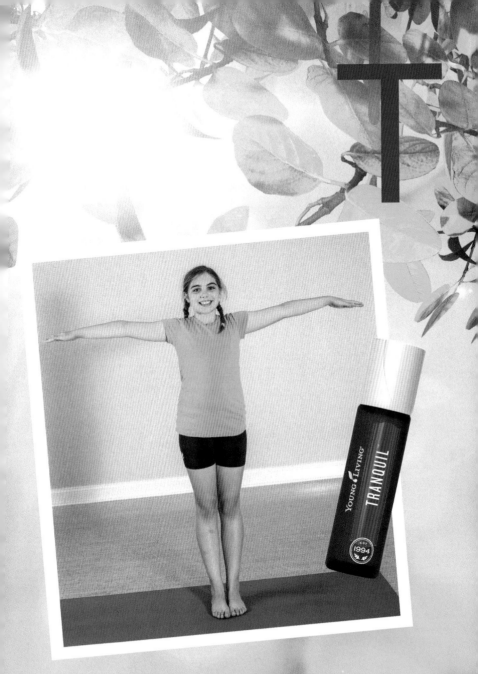

I feel tranquil.

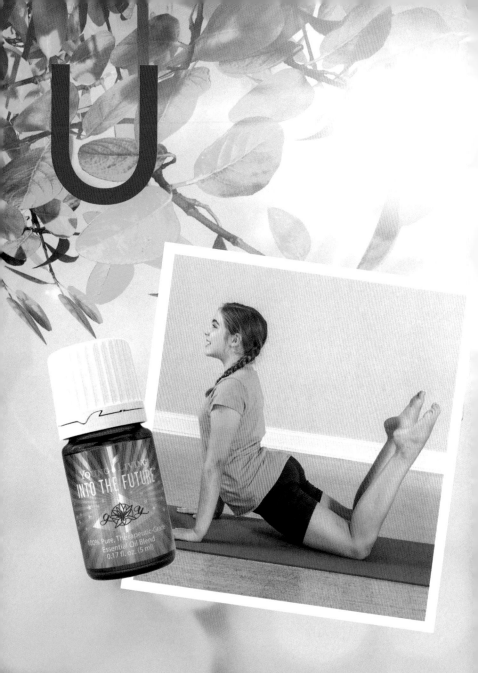

I see into the fUture.

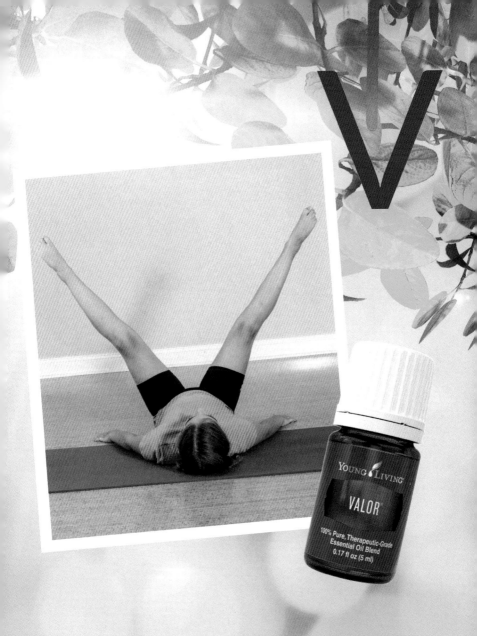

I choose valor.

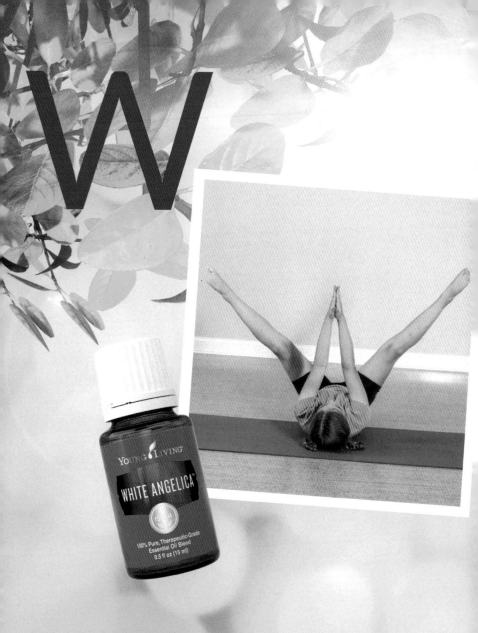

W

WHITE ANGELICA

I feel angelic.

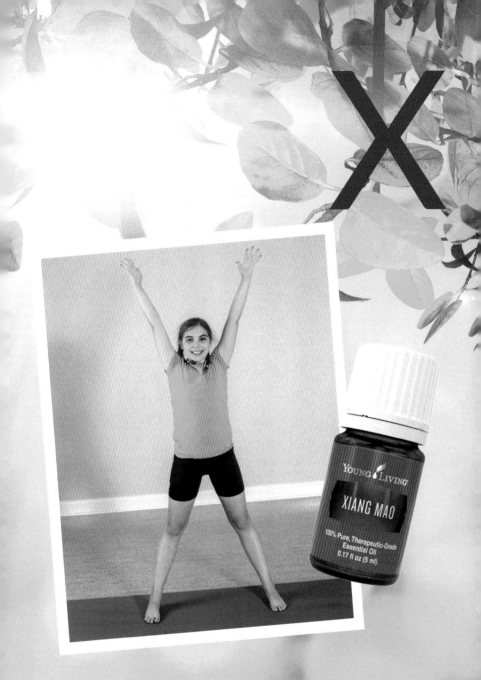

X

Xiang Mao supports me.

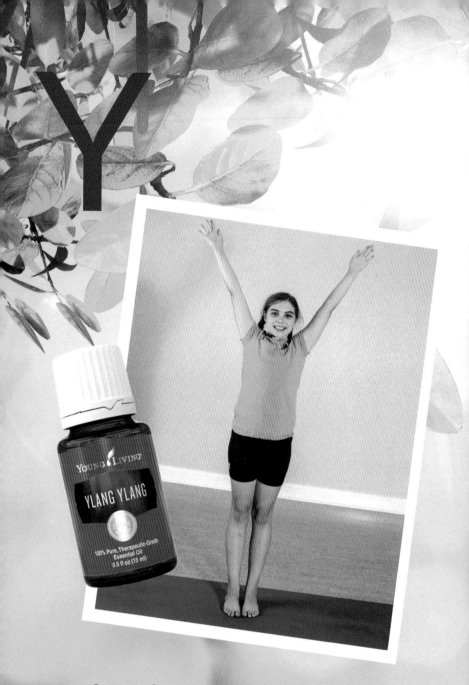

I enjoy ylang ylang.

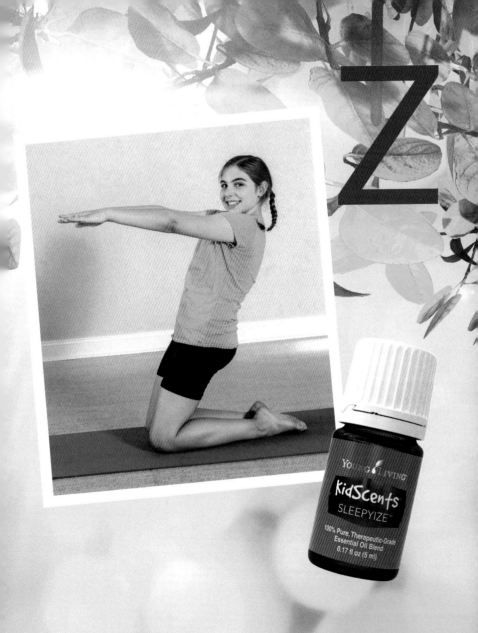

I rest my sleepy eyes.

Alphabet Adventures

Day Plan

In the morning, spell out your main activities of your day – school, music, sports, homework, etc., using the Yoga Alphabet. What are your morning oils you apply?

Name Know-How

Spell your name with your Yoga Alphabet! Make up an affirmation that starts with each letter of your name.

> P – Pampering myself feels good!
> A – I Accept myself!
> M – Make today amazing!

What essential oils come to mind with these affirmations? How about Acceptance™ essential oil? Yes!

Study Buddy

When you are studying, there may be some things you are having trouble remembering. Or, there may be some facts that are really important to recall. This is a great time to use the oils of BrainPower™, Peppermint, or Clarity™ while spelling out the words you are working to remember.

Playtime

We invite you to get silly and creative with the Yoga Alphabet! Put it into your play time and make up games of your own using the letters, your essential oils, and affirmations. There are many more oils to pair with the letters and affirmations. Have fun!

Radical Gratitude

Perhaps there are some things you are radically grateful for and you would like your body, mind, and heart to remember them. Spell them out with our Yoga Alphabet! Examples: Mommy, Daddy, your dog's name, school, your teachers name, etc. As you spell out your Radical Gratitude words, inhale Young Living's Gratitude™ essential oils.

Spell out the crops you would find on Young Living farms. Learn how to spell the names of the farms using your Yoga Alphabet and the states or countries they are in. Use the oils that come from the plants/trees that grow on that particular farm. Example: Spell out Lavender (spell it) in France (spell it) on our farm - Simiane-la-Rotonde (spell it).

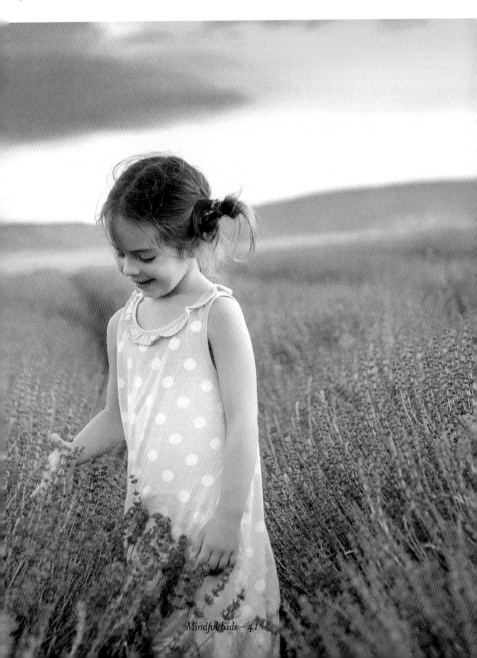

Restful Night

Moving your body at night actually prepares you for a restful night. Before bedtime, spell out 1 – 3 things in your day that you loved. With each word you are spelling, add a restful essential oil such as, Lavender, Sleepylze™, Peace & Calming™, Rutavala™ Roll-on, or Palo Santo.

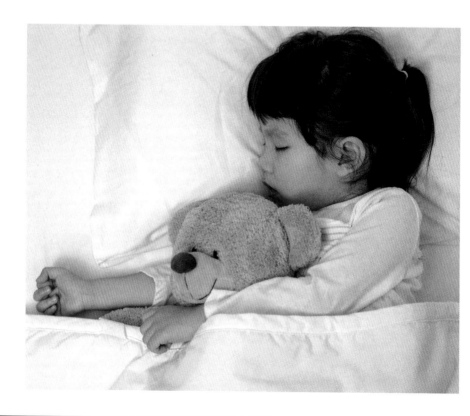

Worldly Awareness – Where in the World?

Learn your states, capital cities, countries, etc., using your Yoga Alphabet for memory recall. Smell an essential oil before you start, while you are studying, and afterwards to help you recall.

Vowels & Consonants

Teach your children to identify the consonants and the 5 vowels in the alphabet. As a reminder, vowels are a, e, i, o, u and sometimes y and consonants are all the other letters in the alphabet. Sing out the vowels while making the shape of the vowel. What essential oil will you pair with this fun ABC play?

Play with More Affirmations

Choose an affirmation that speaks to you. Connect with your favorite essential oil and enhance the effect of its application while you apply it, saying your affirmation using the topical method.

We invite you to be creative and feel your affirmation and oil combo while spelling out how it makes you feel using the Yoga Alphabet.

Here are some examples of our favorite affirmations and essential oils combos.

1) *I am beautiful, bountiful, and blissful.*
   Inhale or apply the oil of Abundance™.

2) *I am happy and free.*
   Inhale or apply the oil of Joy®.

3) *I am love.*
   Inhale or apply the oil of Sacred Frankincense™.

4) *I am peace.*
   Inhale or apply the oils of Peace & Calming™.

Have fun spelling these words with your Yoga Alphabet:

1) Blissful

2) Free

3) Love

4) Peace

If you love this, you will also love our Mindful Meditations Book.
https://www.discoverlsp.com/mindful-meditation.html

Affirmations are a repetition of positive words, sounds, or phrases providing a focused intention and vibration. The sounds of your voice vibrates throughout the entire body. Sound travels efficiently through water. The human body is over 70% water, an excellent conductor for sound and vibration. Affirmations may quiet the mind, and may help bring positive changes within. When words or phrases are spoken out loud, they may encourage and uplift the person speaking them. They bring you into present moment as the brain does not communicate in future or past tense. Let's have some fun with affirmations and ABC's!

Mindful Parents
ABC's & Essential Oils

Children learn the Yoga ABC's while at play! Integrating essential oils while making the shapes of the ABC's stimulates language learning and memory recall. Parent involvement in the language learning process supports your child's development. The ABC's are the essential building blocks and foundation for the English language like the elements of carbon, hydrogen, and oxygen are the building blocks for essential oils and all life on planet Earth. The layering of Yoga ABC's with essential oils supports the foundation to enhance verbal, physical, and emotional communication.

Yoga ABC's & Essential Oils with Kids may support:
* mindful, structured physical activity
* freedom in the whole body, joints and muscles
* verbal communication
* positive body image
* self confidence
* family bonding
* connecting body and mind
* spatial awareness
* emotional intelligence
* memory recall

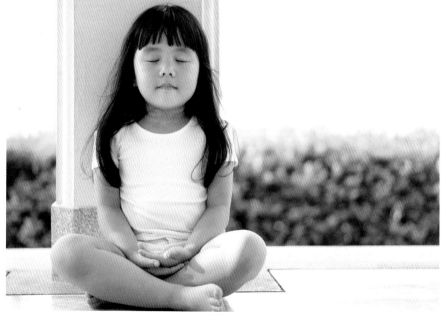

Parents Focus on Positive Reinforcement

Children learn naturally through play and positive reinforcement. Positive Reinforcement is very important to elevate our kid's self-esteem. There is a skill in offering such praise. Using the words, "good boy and/or good girl" are very limiting and do not tell your child the specifics of what they did well. "Good job" is another form of this without being gender specific. While this is a step in the right direction with praise, it is best to curb your "good jobbing." "Good job" loses all meaning if you say it after every letter. Offer specific feedback such as, "Wow, Dakota, you have created the shape of the letter D for your first name! Your body looks so cool!"

Parents, observe how much positive reinforcement you give your children and the style you use. In our experience, behavior can be retrained with specific positive reinforcement efforts with details and authenticity. Then notice how much you ignore. Are you ignoring the good behavior and giving attention to the bad? Let's switch that up and give more attention to the good and ignore the bad. The Yoga Affirmation Alphabet is a fun activity to practice this parenting style.

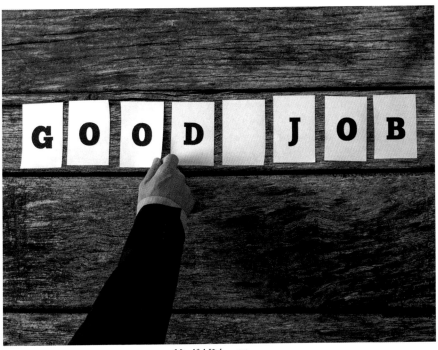

Essential Oils and the Limbic System

We created this book to be a playful and successful tool for parents to teach their children the ABC's with the inhalation of essential oils. They absorb and process new information about the world around them through their senses. Activating a child's sense of smell while learning the basic building blocks of the English language activates the limbic system of the brain that supports memory, communication skills, and emotional health.

The limbic system contains the most basic, life-sustaining and meaningful roles of all brain structure. The limbic system controls emotions, memory, learning, and perceives sensory information. The hippocampus is part of the entire limbic system. The hippocampus helps us form and retain memories, which is very important for learning and development.

Functions of the hippocampus include:
- Forming short-term and long-term memories
- Learning new skills from positive reinforcement
- Sense of direction
- Spatial memory
- Olfaction (smelling) and linking together smells with specific memories

Our sense of smell is unique compared to our other senses (such as taste, sight and hearing) because it bypasses parts of the brain that other types of sensory information often cannot. The aromatic molecules of the essential oils interact with sensors in your nasal cavity, lungs, and pores that easily absorb into the bloodstream, and travel directly through the blood/brain barrier very quickly. Essential oils easily absorb into the bloodstream and cross the blood/brain barrier because our cells recognize that the essential oils contain the same life energy of carbon, hydrogen, and oxygen found in a majority of our human body.

Ever wonder why certain smells conjure up memories and even physical feelings so vividly? Smells may induce emotional reactions based on memories. Smells may transport us back to past memories within moments, invoking a wide range of feelings based on these past events, whether or not we are aware of the source of these feelings.

The limbic system gathers information from the environment through sensory information. For example, the smell of lemon transports me to my grandma's backyard garden in California where I picked the lemons from her lemon tree that I brought inside to her kitchen. I fondly remember her slicing lemons for the sun tea that naturally brewed outdoors all day on her back porch from the sun's rays. I feel love and affection for the memory of my grandma, and I feel sadness at the same time because she no longer is alive.

This story inspired by Stacey's trips to her grandparents in the the Summer.

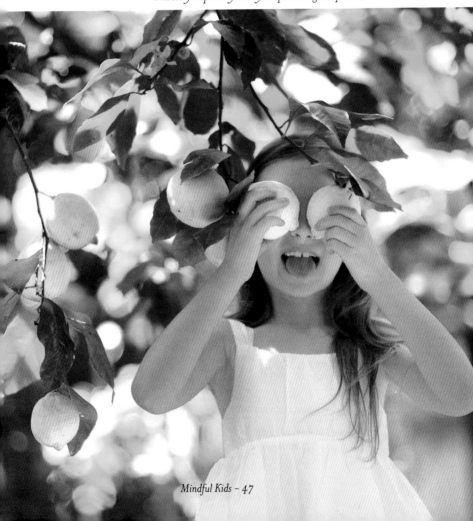

Parents, imagine your child as an adult inhaling the Young Living essential oil of Harmony and remembering learning the alphabet with you as a young child spelling out the letter H with their body and saying the affirmation, "I live in Harmony." You are creating powerful and positive memories with your child.

"I've learned that people will forget what you said, people will forget what you did, but people will never forget how you made them feel."
~ Maya Angelou

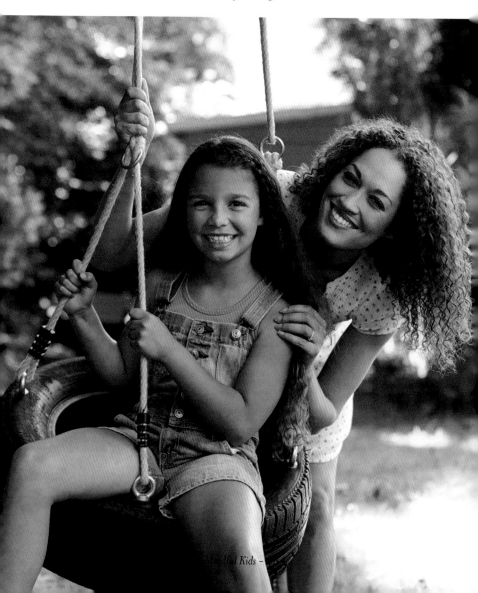

Listen to Your Kids

After you practice the *Yoga Affirmation ABC's,*
What are your kids' affirmations?

_____

_____

_____

_____

_____

_____

How are you feeling? Do you have a favorite game?

_____

_____

_____

_____

_____

What are your favorite essential oils to use with your Yoga Alphabet?

_____

_____

_____

_____

_____

Meet the Authors...

Pamela Hunter and Stacey Vann have been teaching yoga together since 1999 and experiencing Young Living Essential Oils since 2002. We have been using the Yoga Affirmation Alphabet with our own children and children in our yoga classes since 2002.

Founder of Fun Lovin' Wellness, Pamela Hunter believes in awakening awareness and opening paths. Pamela's journey has inspired her and many others to learn and practice self-care. Pamela creates community through her love and education as a Diamond Leader for Young Living Essential Oils sharing "little bottles of love." She has taught yoga since 2001 and is e-RYT 500, Certified YogaKids® Teacher, a Certified UZIT (Urban Zen Integrative Therapy) Trainer and Internationally Respected Integrative Health Coach. She is also certified in several mindful modalities: Clinical Aromatherapy, Spiritual Healing, Reiki, and Reflexology. She is the author of 3 publications - Rise & Shine: 6 Master Steps to Get Moving, Mindful Breathing, and Mindful Meditations. She resides in Chicago area with her husband. Her two grown sons are in college. Pamela is traveling, teaching retreats and workshops, writing, and still growing!
www.FunLovinWellness.com

"Through Awareness, we transform our body and our mind to meet our soul." ~ Pamela Hunter

Stacey Vann, E-RYT500 began teaching yoga in 1997 and started her journey with Young Living in 2002. She weaves and shares the transformative and integrative path of yoga, sound, and Young Living Essential Oils in the U.S. and internationally. Stacey's teaching style is infused with laughter, energy, and love. She encourages her students to attain wellness, joy and connection with a commitment to daily practice, self-care, and an attitude of gratitude. Stacey has 2 publications, Mindful Breathing and Mindful Meditations. Stacey Vann is a mother, Life Coach, doula, reflexologist, Young Living essential oil educator and founder of the Mahabhuta Yoga Festival, co-founder of Galactic Child Yoga, and is co-owner of Breathe Yoga and Wellness Center where she leads 200 & 300-hour teacher training programs in Pensacola, Florida.

"Breathe Deeply, Move Freely, & Live Joyfully." ~ Stacey Vann

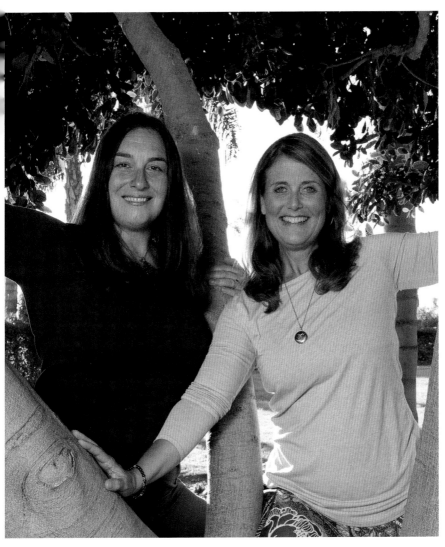

The Yoga ABC's was created 20 years ago by Stacey Vann and is finally being shared in this book. The Yoga ABC's is highlighted in the Galactic Child Yoga Teacher Training. www.galacticchildyoga.com

References

"Elements for Kids."
Ducksters Educational Site, Technological Solutions, Inc,
www.ducksters,com/science/chemistry/hydrogen.php.

"Elements for Kids."
Ducksters Educational Site, Technological Solutions, Inc,
www.ducksters,com/science/chemistry/ecosystems/carbon_cycle.php.

"Elements for Kids."
Ducksters Educational Site, Technological Solutions, Inc,
www.ducksters,com/science/chemistry/oxygen.php.

Young, Gary. Essential Oils Desk Reference.
6th ed. N.p.: Life Science, 2014. Print.

Young Living | World Leader in Essential Oils | Young Living Essential Oils.
Web. 02 Dec. 2014.

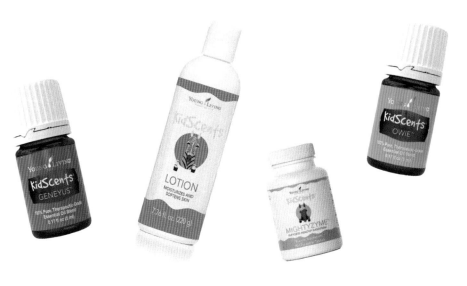

Check out all the
KidScents® Products!

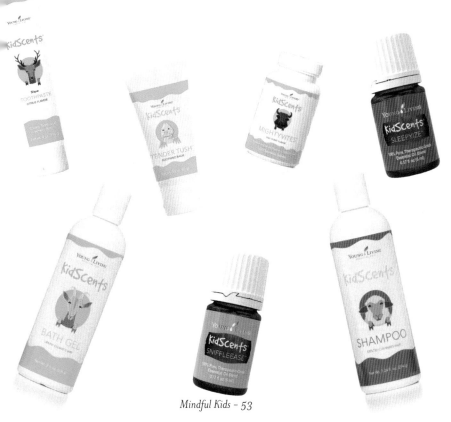